HOME WORKOUT FOR BEGINNERS

The Ultimate Home Workout Training Guide

(How Your Home Workout Plan Can Improve Your Social Skills)

Patrick Dubin

Published by Harry Barnes

Patrick Dubin

All Rights Reserved

Home Workout for Beginners: The Ultimate Home Workout Training Guide (How Your Home Workout Plan Can Improve Your Social Skills)

ISBN 978-1-77485-218-7

Legal & Disclaimer

The information contained in this book is not designed to replace or take the place of any form of medicine or professional medical advice. The information in this book has been provided for educational and entertainment purposes only.

The information contained in this book has been compiled from sources deemed reliable, and it is accurate to the best of the Author's knowledge; however, the Author cannot guarantee its accuracy and validity and cannot be held liable for any errors or omissions. Changes are periodically made to this book. You must consult your doctor or get professional medical advice before using any of the suggested remedies, techniques, or information in this book.

Upon using the information contained in this book, you agree to hold harmless the Author from and against any damages, costs, and expenses, including any legal fees potentially resulting from the application of any of the information provided by this guide. This disclaimer applies to any damages or injury caused by the use and application, whether directly or indirectly, of any advice or information presented, whether for breach of contract, tort, negligence, personal injury, criminal intent, or under any other cause of action.

You agree to accept all risks of using the information presented inside this book. You need to consult a professional medical practitioner in order to ensure you are both able and healthy enough to participate in this program.

TABLE OF CONTENTS

INTRODUCTION...1

CHAPTER 1: THE CHALLENGES OF TRAINING AT HOME......4

CHAPTER 2: FULL BODY STRETCHING EXERCISES AND ITS BENEFITS...8

CHAPTER 3: DO IT YOURSELF...22

CHAPTER 4: HOME WORKOUT ROUTINES - YOUR KEY TO HEALTH AND FITNESS...29

CHAPTER 5: HOW TO WORKOUT AT HOME.....................43

CHAPTER 6: WHAT'S BODYWEIGHT? 47

CHAPTER 7: HOME & CLASSES OR GYM...........................53

CHAPTER 8: THE 3 KEYS OF FITNESS................................61

CHAPTER 9: THE SCIENCE OF WEIGHT LOSS.....................84

CHAPTER 10: THE LIST OF BODYWEIGHT TRAINING EXERCISES 91

CHAPTER 11: WORKOUT 104

CHAPTER 12: HOW TO ENSURE YOUR SAFETY AND GET FAST RESULTS...115

CHAPTER 13: OTHER TIPS FOR A FULL BLAST HOME WORKOUT.. 119

CHAPTER 14: ROWERS... 123

CHAPTER 15: SITTING & STANDING BAND EXERCISES.... 128

CONCLUSION... 139

Introduction

Obesity has been an increasing concern over the years. It's not only about how unattractive your stomach looks. It's also about the serious health effects of extra fat. Even a few extra pounds could lead to multiple health issues such as diabetes, hypertension and heart disease. Unfortunately, there are too many people in our world who don't know or care enough about these issues.

I'm here to assist and tell you that even if your weight is a little bit higher than normal, there are still ways to lose it. You can quickly lose weight and get in form.

I will share a few steps that will help you get the shape you desire. There are many ways to lose fat by lifting weights. However, we want to take things one step further and move in a fast lane. We want fast results. To achieve this, we have created other methods. They will provide you with the best results in a short time by being combined.

Before we begin, I'd like you to know a few things to keep in your mind as we move forward together on this weight loss journey.

Change your diet. This is much simpler than you might imagine. You can start preparing for success by simply listing the new "diet meals" on your grocery lists.

Eat a lot more fruits and vegetables. They have amazing health benefits. You can enjoy the delicious taste of vegetables, in addition to their energy and nutrition.

Get adequate fluids throughout a day. Drink plenty of water. Don't ever feel thirsty. Your body will tell you when you feel thirsty.

Walking when you can is the best option. Even though it might seem tempting to get in your car or take an Uber, walking will be more efficient. Walking matters, and it can be made into a social experience.

Do not go to bed too early. Your body will be more relaxed if you get enough sleep. You'll feel refreshed and ready make it to the next day by sleeping 7-9 hours a night.

Final note: I want you to know that you are investing in your health and well-being by actively moving forward with this book. If you like this book, please let us know via our Facebook page.

http://on.fb.me/1ORuso9

We appreciate you allowing us to help with your fitness goals. I hope you get the most out of what is already inside.

PS.

If you don't have a kindle you can skip to the next chapter or table of contents.

Chapter 1: The Challenges of

Training at Home

What are the problems of training at home? Nothing could be simpler than staying in shape while you have a bench press right at your house.

It's not as easy as it seems. That's why most people start at a gym. Simply stocking up your home with everything you need is the first step. It's possible for bodyweight training to help you get in shape. We'll talk more about that later. It's important to remember that equipment is necessary for quick muscle building results. It means dumbbells. Pull up bars. Bench presses. Treadmills. All of these items cost a lot and take up a lot space.

There is another issue: knowledge. Many people don't know the best ways to train at home. Without a gym, it is difficult to build large muscle. A simple attempt at lifting a barbell yourself in the privacy of your own home could lead to a slipped disk, or even buckled knees. Fear is going to cause immobilization for many people in this regard and stop them from getting into shape.

A lot of people struggle with motivation. If you are trying to get in shape in the front room, then you should avoid TV distractions. It is also important that you stay motivated, even though you may be lying down.

But this isn't always the hardest part...

Pushing yourself from Home

The problem is that you must be able to push your limits in order build strength and fitness. If you are looking to build muscle then you must be able to tear it apart and inject your muscles in metabolites. More on this later. This is easier when you can lift big weights and then reduce your effort each time you succeed. You will find it easier to follow a trainer's instructions. It's much easier to exercise when you're surrounded with people who are hard at work, have no distractions, and have a comfortable floor that's easy to sweat on.

The same goes for losing weight. How do I lose weight? Cardio. It should be high volume and of high intensity. Training is about pushing yourself to the limit, no matter how long you run or how intense your HIIT workouts are.

If you are not at home, it is likely that you will not know how to do these things, or have the necessary equipment.

This book can change all of that. These chapters will help you understand how to quickly build muscle and change your metabolism, all from the comforts of your own home. Once you understand the logic, the key to unlocking the code will allow you to build the power and health of your dreams.

Let's get to it!

Chapter 2: Full Body stretching

exercises and its benefits

Are you aware that stretching should be done before, during and after your workouts. Many people don't pay enough attention. Why? It's because there are no visible results, unlike running, lifting, and any other form of exercise.

Stretching can be great for your health. It will improve your posture and help prevent injuries. It can help boost self-confidence and improve your outlook on life.

Warming up is good for your body and blood flow. Stretching properly can help improve posture and decrease pain after a workout.

Stretching has many advantages

Here are some great benefits to stretching.

It can increase your flexibility.

It corrects your posture and lengthens tight muscles that may not be in their desired position.

It helps to reduce the likelihood of injury during your exercise.

It increases the amount of nutrients and blood in your system.

It reduces muscle soreness.

It prepares you mentally for your main work out.

It reduces stress and tension by relaxing the muscles.

It helps to reduce the risk of muscle cramps.

Make it a Habit

Here are some tips to help make stretching a habit.

Stretch when calm and relaxed

Stretching before and afterwards can help reduce tension.

When you are stretching, remember to take a deep breath.

Hydration is key to flushing out tension and stress released after stretching.

Stretching at the same time every day is a good idea.

Neck Stretching

Our first exercise is going to be on the neck. Stretching your neck muscles increases your range and motion, and can help you to become more flexible. You can also enjoy a number of psychophysiological benefits. These include helping you to relax and de-stress. Regular stretching can prevent tension headaches from occurring.

Maintain a natural position, feet slightly apart, back straightened, and arms at your side.

As though you were looking towards the other side, position your body forward. Hold this for five seconds.

REST – Revert to your starting position and allow yourself to relax for two seconds.

Then repeat the two previous steps in the opposite direction.

Slowly tilt your neck to one side so you feel a bit of tension on the muscle outside. Tend for five seconds.

REST

Continue the previous steps, but now bend in the opposite way, first forwards, then reverses.

Repeat this five times in each direction - look left to right, bend left to right, bend right, bend forwards, and bend backwards.

Finish five repetitions. Perform a few slow roll of the neck to remove any kinks.

Chest Stretches

Your chest stretches increase the flexibility of your shoulders and pectoral (chest), muscles and allow for more motion. They are good for your posture and prevent slouching. Slouching is caused by tight muscles that make it difficult for your shoulders to rest comfortably.

Place your hands behind your head, and stand straight.

Move your hands toward the ground in a pull motion. Push your chest out until you feel some tension in the shoulders and chest.

For 10 seconds, hold this position before returning to your original location.

You can take a break for five seconds.

All steps should be repeated five times.

After you've completed five repetitions, gently roll your shoulders to release any tension.

Single Arm Triceps Stretches

Your triceps is the muscle that runs along the back part of your upperarm. Its job is to extend (straighten out) your elbows. They are important for strengthening your arm and shoulder.

Place your hands on the floor and stand straight with your knees bent.

You can raise one hand and lay your palm on the base your neck.

The opposite hand should be held up towards your elbow. Use it to pull your elbow so that you feel tension in the triceps.

Keep this position for ten second before returning to the original.

Do the same for your opposite arm.

For both arms, repeat the exercise three times.

You can do three repetitions of this exercise. Now, bend your arms slowly and straighten them several time to get rid any kinks.

Shoulder Stretches

Your shoulders are one the most important joints, but they are also fragile. Neglecting to exercise, putting too much pressure on your shoulders, and not taking proper care of them can cause dislocations. Stretching your shoulders will make your muscles flexible and less likely be to place too much pressure upon the joints. This will help reduce the chances of dislocations.

Keep your posture natural.

With one arm raised, place the other parallel to ground. Keep the shoulder straight.

Then, cross your arm across your chest with your other hand and pin it down. To pull the arm back into your chest, use the other hand. You can hold this position for ten minutes before you return to the beginning.

Give yourself five seconds to relax.

Then repeat the same procedure with the other arm.

You should do the exercise three more times for each arm.

To get rid of any kinks, continue to do three repetitions. Swing your arms slowly, in large circles.

Torso Tilts

Your spine is the structural support for your entire body weight. It always bears a load no matter where you are - whether you're standing, sitting or lying down. Because it protects the spinal cord, it is more vulnerable to injury. It is essential to maintain a healthy spine. For this reason, the next three stretches focus on strengthening and flexibility of the muscles that support your spine.

Torso tilts focus on your obliques (muscles along your abdomen's sides) and your pelvic muscle, increasing their ability to stabilize your spine.

Place your hands on your chest and keep your back straight.

Take a 2-2-4kg dumbbell and hold it in your hand. The dumbbell does not serve as a strength training tool. Its sole purpose is to stabilize your exercise motion, keeping your arm straight and pointing downward.

Slowly, tilt your pelvis in order to hold the dumbbell. Once the dumbbell has the arm perpendicular, the dumbbell will naturally move the arm. Until tension is felt on the opposite end, To counterbalance this, gently swing your opposite hand upwards. Tend this position for ten seconds before gently returning to a straight position.

Switch the dumbbells to the opposite hand and repeat the process for the other side.

Repeat this three times on both sides.

You can finish three repetitions and then lower the dumbbell. Perform slow pelvis roll to get rid of kinks.

Back compressions

Back compressions strengthen the stability of the spine by focusing on the many muscles involved in its anchoring. Because of this, they are some of the most important stretches to do.

You will need to get down on your hands, knees and knees so that your arms and thighs are parallel to the ground.

Slowly curve the spine inward. Do this until your back is as concave, and tension begins to build along your spine. Continue to hold for five seconds and then return to the original position.

You can take a break for 2 seconds.

Slowly curve outward your spine, making sure your back is as convex and straight as you can. To achieve the best curvature, slide your hands forward and bend your knees. Hold the position for five second, then return to the starting position.

You can take a break for 2 seconds.

Alternate between curling outward and inward until five times.

Do a series of deep bows when you are done. This will get rid any kinks.

Lower Back Twist

This exercise will stretch the lower back muscles as well and glutes. If you spend your day sitting down, this exercise will be especially beneficial. This can lead you to back pain, poor posture, and other health issues.

Sit straight up with your legs straight in front.

Bend one knee and cross the other leg over the bent foot.

Bend your torso toward the bent leg. Now, twist your torso so that your opposite elbow is against the bent knee.

You can now twist your torso to the limit by using the elbow. Hold for five second and relax for a further two.

Repeat five times.

You can return to the starting position by bringing the other leg up. Repeat the exercise for five more times.

You can finish the exercise by standing up with your feet straight out. Then, twist your torso to stretch your kinks.

Double Leg Curl Back

Your legs do a lot of work every day. A slight loss of strength or flexibility could have a significant impact on your overall wellbeing. It is possible to get hurt, sprains, or tears from your legs, joints, and muscles. This can be prevented by stretching your legs regularly.

Double-back leg curls are good for stretching your front quadriceps. They improve the flexibility of the knee by allowing it bend further for longer periods.

Your front should be flat on the floor. Keep your head elevated by using your forearms. Do not elevate your upper torso.

Place your feet on your back and bend your knees.

You can feel the tension in your spine by arching your back. This position should be held for 10 seconds. Then, return to your starting point.

Give yourself five seconds to relax.

Repeat the above five times.

For kinks to be worked out, you can stand up and perform several back-kicks each leg.

Stretching is essential for both beginners and for experienced hands. You can start stretching daily if you are just starting out.

Try stretching at least for a week before starting your 30-day workout challenge. The positive changes you see from stretching compound over time, so they are more visible over time. If you complete the 30-day challenge, your flexibility will be increased and you'll have the stamina and endurance to resist the temptation of giving up.

Chapter 3: Do It Yourself

The rise of social media makes it easy to connect with many people from all walks of the world. It is much easier to find ways to fit in the crowd, because you don't want your ideas to be rejected. This can also impact your homework plan. To win the acceptance of others, you might be looking to lose weight. This chapter discusses how to get your life on track by making it all about yourself.

Avoid unnecessary attention

It's not what you want, for people to pay unnecessarily attention to your physique. Unfortunately, many people are living with this reality, especially plus-size ones. Many people are mocked for being overweight by the movies and internet. In fact, excess weight is not good. Excessive weight is not good for your health and can make you look worse. The wrong way to start your workout program is not a good idea. It's okay to lose weight. But, you shouldn't start your workout plan on the wrong note. Remember, muscle building and weight loss is a gradual process. The vision you have should be able to visualize your ideal body. However, accepting yourself is key to achieving your goals.

Be a person you can be proud of, and someone who has earned the love and respect from others. If you find that your friends often make insensitive remarks about your appearance, you need not be close to them. Don't be embarrassed to be yourself, even if you want to improve.

Good friends will be able to point out your faults and offer a roadmap to rectify them. They will support you in your efforts and provide moral support. It doesn't mean that people won't make fun of your efforts to lose weight and build muscles. Insensitive people will always find a reason to mock you, regardless of your achievements. Cristiano Ronaldo is the greatest soccer player ever, yet people still make demeaning comments about him. You can learn to love and accept yourself no matter what your appearance.

Maintaining Fitness with the Right Motivation

Authors of fitness books and articles will often encourage people use their worst experiences and negative comments to inspire them. For example, if you were a woman who was dumped by your boyfriend for being overweight, they might encourage you to look more attractive to him. It sounds great on the surface. You might imagine going out on an intimate date with another guy and posting the image on social networks. This is a sign you're insecure.

Do not waste your time on someone who has a bad body. It's different if you are not willing to work hard to improve your appearance. It is not right for a guy to hook up with another woman because he thinks you are less sexy. It is the exact same for a lady that breaks up with her man because of the same reasons. The worst thing you could do is start to visit the gym and/or begin a training program in revenge.

You will eventually feel discouraged and frustrated if you begin exercising to prove your point. Look at it this way: even when their spouse is beautiful, some guys cheat on her. This is what many famous people think about. As with women who are attractive, men who have attractive bodies lose their partners. This is why physical appearance does not matter. If you love someone, they will always be there for you no matter how thin or slender you are. They might encourage weight loss, but not by making threats to swap you for someone slimmer.

Stay clear of the media pressure

Some people recognize the source of stress. For instance, your boss may have been frustrating recently. Either way, it is possible that you have been unhappy with your spouse or children in the past. The truth is that media influences can make you feel bad. A negative comment on a picture can lead to you feeling unhappy about your body.

Many people post highly edited photos in order to receive likes and positive remarks. You may be thinking that these people are living better lives than you. In reality, they're just living a lie. Before you do any thing, ask yourself what the motive is. You may be looking to get more likes on social networks. You might choose to be called hot or sexy, gorgeous or handsome.

These comments can actually be very helpful and can bring you joy. However, you may feel let down or rejected if someone calls you ugly or fat. You can be desperate and try to prove someone wrong. It's not possible to sustain this. They might mock you for your efforts to improve.

Don't post photos or videos until you have the body you want before encouraging others. Post them only to show your detractors you're making improvements. You may be ridiculed by your detractors, which can only lower your self-esteem. To get back in control of your lives, you may need to be away from digital life. This is called digital detox. For more information, see "Disconnect to reconnect" by this author.

Signs you are working for the wrong reasons

You can tell when your motivation to start a gym is wrong. It will influence the way you do things. You should examine your motives and method.

* Impatience can cause you to work too hard

*You indulge in too many types of movements. Your body feels swollen and irritable, and pain may last up to a week. *You are experiencing pain on only one side.

These signs are common among people who are trying make a point. This can lead to a fixation on one side of the body and not your overall health. You'll feel desperate and will try too hard.

Chapter 4: Home workout routines -

Your key to health and fitness

Home exercise is becoming mainstream. WebMD reports that 63% American grownups are overweight/fat. This shows that there is a need to ensure our well-being. Due to the hectic schedules of our families and work, we are unable to make time for exercise. It's important to discover great home workouts.

Everyone should be fit and young. We as a society recognize that this requires effort and some investment. Let's begin with the basics. We as a community know that there are no easy ways to get thinner. It takes effort, nutrition, and movement. That's the best way to properly lose weight and keep it off. Make sure you take care of your body and get a decent home-wellness plan. This will help you live a healthy lifestyle. It should be transformed into a "Way of life".

What are the best home exercise routines?

By simply walking after supper every night, or during the mid-day break at your workplace, you can improve your health. This may seem impossible for some people. The majority of home exercise projects can be accomplished by using a quality DVD. You have probably seen the infomercials from Insanity (or P90X) and 10 Minute Train. These are excellent home exercise plans for most people. However, which one is right? This is the most important thing you should know. You need a home fitness program that will keep you motivated and make you smile. Recall, it should be a way to live so that you can keep making progress in weight loss or improving your overall health.

Do you like to move? Or maybe you're a secondary or competitor school. Perhaps this is the first time that you've tried any type or activity. There are many home workouts that can help. Perhaps you have an active schedule. There are plenty of home exercise programs for you. You don't have to excuse yourself. It's time to be honest with yourself and take charge of your health and well-being.

One of the greatest things about a decent home workout is that they are very affordable. Many dollors per year will be required to participate in an exercise club. A decent exercise DVD will only cost you $40-$120. The DVDs can be used for long periods of time and have different degrees force.

3 Steps for Success

I believe there are 3 key steps you can take to create a productive home exercise program.

1. Make a commitment to your well-being and wellness. In the event that you don't see the value in it, no one else will. Find your "WHY". Your "WHY" is what you need

to do. You might have health reasons, disappointment with the way you live now or any other reason.

2. Focus on a particular program. There are many home exercise plans to choose from. The right one is for you.

3. Backing-It has been proven that a larger percentage of people who want to lose weight are more likely to succeed if they are being supported or in a care program.

Once these 3 steps are completed, you'll be well on your way to great wellbeing. This will ultimately lead to your Success. To lose weight, you do not need to go to the gym or join a local wellness center. You can now get decent exercise at home. Make the commitment to get started on your home exercise plan today.

The Easy Way to Stay Motivated: Home Workout Routines

You know a few home workouts you should do. You have enough space. You have everything a home fitness center could need. You're willing to get active. You will be fit and strong. The women, or the men as the case may have, will be all over you.

executioner body.

This will allow you to start working out and make it a habit of doing so for the entire week. You might feel a bit sore, but you persevere. You are able to see some positive outcomes from the last week. But at that point, you're exhausted and need to work late. You are so tired that you can't exercise the next morning. You're grumpy, but the next morning comes and your favorite TV series is on. This continues until you realize you aren't the person you think. So dismal.

You may not realize it but you have gained 10 pounds in no time and you are now more confused than ever. Keep in mind that you don't need to be harsh on yourself. Everyone experiences lack of inspiration at some point, even those who are really into exercising. While it's best to never stop exercising, it's okay to have one exercise a day. You don't have to do a lot to get refocused if it is something you can do.

You can remain motivated, regardless of whether your exercise at home is at the rec center or at home. This is the only way to stay persuaded.

1. Ask yourself the following: "Why would I like to be fit as fiddle?"

Being honest with yourself can help you discover the reasons why you need to exercise. You may exercise to feel better, be more attractive to your partner, or be a better competitor. You might be able to explain your reasons.

2. 2.

There is a lot more intensity in the written word, especially when it involves defining an objective. While you don't have to make it a habit of mentioning it every day, it helps if there are self-inspiration problems.

3. Keep track of your personal development with a Training Journal.

One of the best persuasive tools you have is the ability to keep track of how many sets, reps, rest periods, and weight you used. Since I was 15, I have used a preparation diary. Once you notice the improvements in your diary and see what you have done in the mirror to reflect your efforts, it is possible to get energized to work harder in preparation.

4. Utilize a preparation accomplice.

If you're unsure if you can do it all on your own, then get someone else to do it for you. A companion can help you keep track of your preparations and remind you to do them. To help you achieve your wellness goals, a prep accomplice is a wonderful way to get self-motivation. A side benefit to working out with a friend is that it is easier and more enjoyable to do so with another person.

5. 5. Get a personal trainer.

In the event you feel stuck or unable to push yourself, consider hiring a fitness coach. It's both inspirational and good for your wallet to hire a fitness coach. The cost of an instructional course is charged each time that you miss it. Undoubtedly, the greatest ability of a personal trainer is to persuade, to guide you to where you will be able propel. The best way to help people who are truly inspired is to individual prepare.

Take off your handweights and home exercises, and follow these suggestions to stay motivated.

Building your Home Workout Plan

You must exercise. However, you'd prefer to do some kind of home exercise program than go to the rec room.

You also don't need to purchase expensive gym equipment.

You don't need expensive equipment or to go to a gym to get great exercise. You can easily create your very own Home Workout Programs for amazing results.

When I first got into the wellness sector, I attended business rec center and I wasn't disappointed. I looked into it and found home exercise programs that were just as feasible and cost less than I was paying.

You can use the heaviest part of any home exercise routine to lose fat, by using only the largest, most grounded muscles.

You will use the most muscles during an exercise if this happens. It means those muscles will consume a larger amount of calories to recuperate than if it were an exercise done primarily with smaller muscles.

I'll use the pushup as a model. A pushup is a movement that uses your chest, shoulder muscles, rear arms, shoulders, and lower back. It also involves actuating your center, which helps to settle your whole body. Contrast that with the bicep turn. Bicep twist is basically a way to disconnect your biceps and lower arms muscles to lift the weight. It also involves using your shoulders, center and for balance. Is it safe for you to say that you don't use a lot of muscle in the pushup compared to the bicep rotation?

So, it seems that your body will be consuming more calories after the exercise to repair the muscle from the pushups.

We will also begin from that place.

Classifications in Your Workout Routines

There are five basic types of developments that we'll remember when creating home exercise schedules (and here are certain models).

1. Squat – Like a Bodyweight Stairlift

2. Single Leg--a model would make a lurch

3. Pushing Movement. A pushup

4. Hop - like a bouncing jack

5. Center - a board held

Don't let your guard down, though. When building your home exercise program, it is important to start with a full pushup.

For those who are just beginning to exercise, you might start with a pushup on the divider. If that gets easier, you might try doing them on your knees. You can try them again on your feet if that is easier.

Building your Home Workout Routines

We need to organize this now.

Pick one of the exercises from each of these classes. Each one will last 30 seconds.

A tenderfoot would do this.

1. Lying Hip Extension for 30 Seconds

2. Divider Pushup -- 30 seconds

3. Hopping Jacks, 30 seconds

4. Side Leg Raise -- 15 seconds per leg

5. Stooping Plank: 30 seconds

You would perform each of those five activities with no rest between them. After you finished the Kneeling Plank you would rest about 30-60 seconds, then you would repeat the circuit. Rest for 30-60 seconds more, then repeat the process. These activities can be altered to be more challenging if your level is higher or lower.

You could also do a bodyweight push-up or a bodyweight pull-up on your toes.

Pushup on your knees or toes.

It is better to do the burpees or fold hops than the bouncing jumps

You should be able to do the opposite and walk forward, or in a strolling hurry, instead of raising your leg.

A board with a complete board or aboard on a steadiness board instead of the bowingboard

Made for You Home Workouts

You may prefer to create your own home exercises schedules instead.

You may also find other items in my collection that you might like.

Most importantly, you can choose whether to go with a novice, intermediate or advanced program. There is something to suit everyone, whether you are just starting out or you have been training for some time and are looking for something more.

Each of the home exercise routines lasts 90-days. They will let you know what activities to do and how they should be done (with composed, image AND video shows). It takes around 30 minutes to complete each schedule, three days per semaine. A steadiness ball is your most essential gym equipment.

A Fat Loss Nutritional and 7-Minute Abs Guide are included.

A guide on how to create your own home exercise routine

If you follow the steps above, you can create home exercise plans that will work for you.

You could also use a 30-Minute Fitness Workout to save some time. It's easy to lose 10, 15, 20 or more pounds in 90-days. And you don't even need to go out to buy expensive gym equipment.

Chapter 5: How to Workout At Home

You might be fooled if you think you will just unroll your yoga mat and begin a home workout. You'll end up staring at your old, stretched out resistance bands or that dumbbell that doesn't know what to do next.

Know your target.

Number one: Set your goals for your workouts at-home. Are you ready to give up the gym? Want to add convenience to your studio or gym workouts by doing some at-home work outs? This will have an impact on the style and length of the workouts you do and the equipment needed.

Plan your room space.

Make sure to find a spot that's big enough for at least one mat. This will give you ample space to stretch and do core exercise. Keep your equipment stored under your bed, or your wardrobe, to save space when you're not using it. Based on the type of exercise you choose, you might adjust the settings. HIIT is more difficult and requires a firm floor. Yoga or Pilates can be done anywhere.

Apartment dwellers must be aware of the level of noise. If you are tired of listening to your music on the stereo, consider putting on headphones that don't get stuck to your jumping cord. Then, you won't have the distraction of Lizzo's song "Sweet as Hell", going upstairs to the family and the child. Although you might not feel the need to pound heavy dumbbells into the ground after your last hard rep, or to do jump squats at 2 AM, there are plenty of quieter options. They target the same muscle areas and can be just as rewarding.

Set up a plan.

Don't leave your home at 6 p.m. to go to the gym. Or you might end up watching Netflix and putting off your workouts. It's possible that you could skip your workouts at home. It is possible to create a routine like you would at the gym or in the studio.

If you want to keep your workouts on schedule, it is worth applying the same logic at home. "If someone asks you if you want to meet at five, you should tell them, "Sorry. I have an interview; how about four?"

Keep in mind that no matter where your workouts take you, consistency will be key to your success. Stephanie Howe is an ultrarunner at CLIF Bar and has a PhD from nutrition and exercise science.

"This will help you to move forward, not stagnate." You can ask these questions to help you figure out the best way for your home to incorporate your workouts.

* Are you more motivated to work before dawn or after-work sweat?

* How many hours do you want to dedicate to your homework?

* Would your friends or roommate do it?

* Do you have a child, partner or pet that needs to be taken care of?

* Can you guarantee that your workouts don't hinder your productivity if you're working from home?

* Would you be interested in some encouragement via a fitness app? Or are you already a master of your own workout plan.

* Are you looking to get sweaty? (If the answer is "drenched", you may find a 20-minute lunch break workout not the best.

Chapter 6: What's bodyweight?

One of the most beneficial exercises is bodyweight. You don't need to use weights, or any other equipment. Instead, you use your own body weight as resistance during your workouts. Many of you have probably done bodyweight exercise before. Have you ever tried pull-ups, push-ups, or sit ups? That's a good start for bodyweight exercise.

Be sure to include your bodyweight in your daily exercise routine, regardless of whether you are already doing a regular workout. Add a few crunches, lunges, and some other exercises to get you started.

The Health Benefits of Bodyweight Exercises

The obvious benefit of bodyweight exercises is the lack of need to purchase expensive equipment. You can do any bodyweight exercise from your home at any given time. For pull ups, you will need to have a bar installed. However, this is not a costly option if your home has enough space.

Exercises that focus on bodyweight are great for strengthening your muscles and working out. These exercises can help tone, tone, or sculpt your muscles. Depending on which type you choose, you may be able to either build up muscle or do both. The results you get will be amazing.

It's less likely that you will injure or strain yourself while doing bodyweight exercise. And, since you are only working with your weight, it's difficult to push against a heavy weight or pull on someone else.

With the right diet and bodyweight exercises, you can lose weight while toning your body. Bodyweight is the winner, no matter what way you look at this. Let us now see how to do these moves.

Weight loss is key to effective fitness

What you want from exercise will affect how effective your workouts are. Increase the number you do of each rep if you're looking to gain more strength and endurance. If you want to increase your strength and endurance, you could do the exercises in a different style.

Remember that even though your risk is lower than with other types exercise, you still have the potential to injure yourself or cause strain. It is important to warm up and stretch before starting your full exercise routine. You should also end with a cooldown. You should also drink plenty water to stay hydrated. To get the best results, it is important to be consistent. This will make it impossible to get results. Do moderate to hard exercise at least three days a weeks. Try to add some variety on the other days.

Different Muscle Types

To ensure you exercise every muscle group, not just a few, it is crucial to do so. It's important to be able to identify the muscles groups you are trying to target and how best to exercise them.

Upper Body

Biceps located at the front arm - bicep curls

Triceps - These are located at the back end of the arm. Pushups, triceps extension and sips.

Deltoids: Located on your shoulder cap, they are used to do push-ups, bench presses and side or rear arm raises.

Rhomboids, located between the shoulderblades - Chin-ups/bent arm rows

Pectorals – The muscles around your chest. Push-ups, pull-ups.

Trapezius: Located at the top of your back. Upright rows and shoulder shrugs.

Latissimus Dorsi: Located in your middle section of the back. Pull-ups, pulling-downs, and chin ups.

Mid-Section

Abdominals, located in the abdomen. Leg raises and crunches.

Glutes: Located in the buttocks. Leg presses and squats are examples of glutes

Obliques: Located to the side, torso – Crunches

Lower Body

Quadriceps – These are located at the front end of the thighs.

Hamstrings: Located at the back side of the thighs.

Adductors – located on the inner thighs – Worked in conjunction with the glutes

Abductors: Located on the outer Hips.

Erector Spinae (located in the lower right - back extensions

Gastrocnemius & Soleus – Located in back of lower leg – standing and seated calf rises

Chapter 7: Home & Classes Or Gym

For beginners

If you're new to aerobics, it is easy to get overwhelmed by all of the information. There are many options for working out. However, if there is a program that works for you, it will make you much more healthy. Your body needs to move quickly, and your heart must work hard. Don't assume that you have to get there first. Moving up to advanced aerobics takes effort. This may include walking or running in place and performing a number of movements that can be intimidating. Additionally, it is unsafe to begin other than with a beginner as you might hurt yourself.

It is easy to learn aerobics for beginners. The goal is to get your blood flowing. You can start by walking around or running in one place. You can move both your arms up or down. You can move your arms upward and downward. This is the best place to start aerobic training. You can build up your fitness and work up to a good level. You can increase your ability to do more and faster movements.

A second thing you need to keep in mind is the fact that aerobics often works well with music. The best way to do it is to use the music as a motivator and keep your body moving. It's possible to also time your workouts to music. Music can be your motivation and can keep you going.

There are many other options to help you get started, including brisk running, cycling, swimming yoga and Pilates.

Aerobics at Your Home

There are many methods that you can make aerobics more effective for you. First, you must understand how vital aerobic exercise is for your overall health. You can be healthy by simply walking and lifting weights. (If you don't have weights, compromise by eating tins full of carrots or similar. To truly be healthy, you need to get your heart rate up and your blood pumping. Aerobic exercise, which allows you to connect all parts of your body, is crucial for you.

Some people are unable to attend the gym or take classes for their health. Because of their work and family commitments, many people cannot go to the gym.

These places do not work for their schedules.

There are many ways you can exercise at home. As we've already seen, the basic principles of aerobics are to get the heart pumping, and your breathing rate up.

First and foremost, get a bike/treadmill in your home. It can be kept in a central location so you are always ready to go.

Another option is to make a running routine. It can include skipping, running in place and even running around a block. All these are great because you can personalize your workout to meet your needs.

A log, or a diary, should be kept of all your home workouts. This allows you to track your progress and make any adjustments necessary. Prior to starting a new workout, don't exercise within two hours of having had a meal. If you feel faint or lightheaded, it is a sign that you need to stop. If your condition continues to deteriorate, contact a doctor immediately.

Always warm up before starting any exercise. You can start by stretching each muscle. To avoid injury, you must make sure your muscles are warm. To increase your heart rate, you can walk on the spot or do light jogging. Once you have done this, you can start your planned workout. Do some deep, slow breathing and stretches to cool your heart. Keep track of your heartbeats daily in your diary. Then you'll be able to notice the differences.

Aerobic classes

Aerobics will allow you to stay trimmer, be more flexible, and enjoy other physical activities longer. A class can help you stay motivated and will give you the motivation to continue. You can also find people on the same level you are, which will help you not feel intimidated. To be able to enjoy working out, it is crucial that you learn the basics and also master new moves. To help you get the most from your workout, your class instructor should have extensive experience in their area.

We all know that exercise is hard work. You have to motivate yourself to go to the gym, or even get on your bike. By signing up for an aerobics classes, you can make this a regular activity, and it will also help you avoid putting it off. If you don't have the motivation to work out, then maybe a class isn't for you. A class may be better for you.

Personal Trainers

There are many situations in life where you might need the assistance of a personal coach. One such instance is when you do aerobics. You can reach your fitness and maintenance goals much faster with the guidance of a personal trainer. It is not difficult to find the right trainer. However, it is crucial to find one that you feel at ease with and who truly understands your needs. You might find it hard to be happy with a trainer who makes you feel stressed, but this could lead you to becoming dissatisfied and not being your best. Worse yet, you could quit aerobics altogether.

Personal trainers allow you to be fully yourself and still be able do your best. Your trainer can only give you so much help. You are responsible for the results. Your trainer will encourage and support you, but also allow you to work at the pace that suits you.

A personal trainer can motivate you, and help you achieve your goals. This will ensure that you don't put it off for later. It will make you very happy if your trainer is willing and able to help with any concerns you may have.

Aerobic Machines

Aerobics might be easier if you are using a machine, rather than walking, running, and skipping. Aerobics has to be personalized to your body and best for your health. You should work closely with your trainer and physician. They will be able to help you achieve your goals.

The body and the mind.

Machines are becoming very popular for using to exercise. They are easy and simple to use. You don't have worry about weather, or finding the time to exercise. A bike or treadmill are the best and most popular. You can train on these machines regardless of what time it may be or how the weather. You will see results in no time if your heart rate and breathing rate are the same. You can also do it at home, which is much more convenient than visiting the gym. On the flip side, if your gym is accessible, you'll find others and maybe even your personal trainer to encourage you.

Chapter 8: The 3 Keys Of Fitness

These three elements form the so-called "keys of fitness", and you need them all to get any kind of exercise and healthy lifestyle. This program does provide fast results, provided it is respected. But, for long-term success, you will need to put effort into making fitness your lifestyle and not just a solution. We will be discussing all three elements of Training, Nutrition, and Rest. The goal is to give you both the essential knowledge as well as the latest techniques in all three areas in order maximize your results. Training is the fun part.

Training

The most crucial step in building muscle is to train the muscular system. This is because it stimulates your body to grow into a stronger, healthier, and more functional organ. To see results, a training program must be effective. However, as the fitness industry grows exponentially over 30 years, new diets/workout programs, supplements, and ideologies seem to appear almost daily. So before we discuss your workout program let's take a look at what we do know about training. Then we can build on our knowledge. Different types of training became inextricably competitive. With the increase in demand for body-defining activities and bodybuilding techniques, there was a growing market.

We are left to wonder, which is the best kind of exercise? My opinion is that this question has no answer. As each form of exercise has its own advantages and disadvantages, it's impossible to know the right answer. However, this book will give you a clearer picture of the fundamental principles behind the creation of this workout program.

First and foremost, my fitness journey started with bodybuilding. Or, to give you a deeper answer, my parents bought me an annual membership to a local gym and a personal training program. Because my body was not "manly", it didn't seem that my body was going to change anytime soon. Bodybuilding is very effective because it focuses on building size. Each exercise aims to do so by building muscle and compound movements when needed. This is why it is crucial to incorporate bodybuilding principles, exercises and techniques into my workout plan.

Calisthenics is a form of exercise that uses your body's weight and does not require you to join a gym. Calisthenics parks began to emerge, which allow more people to begin working out, even if they don't have to buy a membership. Calisthenics is something I enjoy. Bodyweight exercises make up a large portion of my workouts. Another very important benefit of calisthenics (in my opinion) is the way it burns fat. This is because more compound movements activate muscles and cause them to consume more calories.

Crossfit is often criticized by bodybuilders and calisthenics lovers. I am not surprised. Crossfit trains the muscles and not the muscles. The exercises are executed in a way that allows for more repetitions with a far lower quality. Crossfit is more dangerous than other forms of bodybuilding and calisthenics because it places less tension on the muscles. Crossfit-like workouts I don't recommend because I find them ineffective.

Group training is becoming the second most popular form for exercise. Group training classes provide a cheaper alternative to personal trainers for those looking to lose weight or gain muscle definition. This is because a professional instructs a group of people through a series explosive exercises. Energizing music and atmosphere make the workouts enjoyable and productive. This book provides a workout program that explains the basics of group training.

For the actual routine you will need a set of bodybuilding, calisthenics, and cardio exercises. They are simple to do with little or no equipment. I recommend buying a set with adjustable weight dumbbells, a 5kg kettlebell set, and a jumprope. This is the structure of your workout.

Workout structure

There are three main movements to exercise. These are pulling, pushing, or cardio. All three play an important role in any workout. You will be able to complete our program in the comfort of your own home, and it will take you 5 days a weeks to train.

Monday	Tuesday	Wednesday	Thursday	Friday	Saturday	Sundays
Push	Pull	Leg/Cardio	Rest	Push	Pull	

The push/pull-legs Split is a sophisticated technique that bodybuilders use to train the muscles twice a week. It provides the most stimulus to the fibers. A Push day is three days apart. This allows for fibers and strength to recover and strengthen. The soreness will fade away.

Push days combine exercises for muscles that need to be activated by pushing, such as the chest, shoulders, and triceps.

Pull day follows the same principle, but for the back and biceps. Those muscles require pulling in order strengthen.

Leg exercises require a lot of pushing. But because we are talking mainly about the lower body sore muscles that have not yet regenerated in the upper part of our bodies don't impact training the legs.

Cardio, which is based upon increasing pulse and burning calories, can be done in many different ways. But, with this system cardio becomes simple.

Push Day

Pushups will be the core of any push-day workout. We highly recommend them. The pushup, while it targets your chest, is also a fantastic exercise. As secondary muscles, your shoulders and triceps get engaged. This allows you to increase power output and stability.

These images are a demonstration of how to properly perform the pushup. Start by placing your hands directly below your shoulders. Keep your feet in line with the ground. Slowly lower your body and keep your elbows in line with the ground. The final phase of the exercise is to move your body away the ground and flex your chest muscles and triceps.

The push up will be the most important part of the push day. However, there are many variations. In order to target different parts of the body, variations will be made in the hand positioning as well as the body's alignment to the ground.

To start, let's talk about hand positioning. We have the classic pushup. Your hands are under your shoulders and you find the perfect balance between tension on the chest (and tension on the triceps). The diamond pushup is the next. With the hands placed directly under the chest (its name derives from the shape that the hands make when touching underneath the chest), it primarily targets the quadriceps. Last, but not least, is the wide pushup. This type of pushup relies heavily on hand positioning. Performers position their hands approximately an inch or so outward, increasing distance between them. Wide pushups target the chest more, keeping it under tight tension even when the body tilts upward.

This second variation can be attributed to our body's position relative to the floor. The classic pushup has both the feet and hands on ground, and targets the chest. However, isolation work is usually required for a lower level. The elevation effect is achieved by positioning our arms and feet above the ground. This isolates either the upper section or the lower. If we place our feet at the top of the table, or on a furniture piece, we can do the decline pressup. This allows us to focus on the lower part of the chest.

The second variation on body-positioning is going be the exact opposite to the decline pushup. When our hands are higher than our feet, this gives us the

Incline pushup position

This is the opposite of a decline pushup. The upper chest area can be isolated while the shoulders engage slightly more than the decline.

As an alternative to doing pushups, you can wrap a resistance bracelet around your shoulders and wrap it onto your hands.

Plenty.

The lateral raise is the next big shoulder exercise that we will implement. There is only so much we can do, since the pushup already builds the shoulders. However, push days will heavily rely on various pushup variations.

To do the lateral raise, you will need dumbbells. You can use even one gallon bottles. Because the shoulder's anatomy permits for light weight training, the three major shoulders falls under the "small muscles" category, it is possible to use dumbbells. The lateral elevate requires the user to lift the dumbbells outwards. The lateral elevate is extraordinarily effective. This is achieved by slow, controlled lifting.

The resistance band can be used by placing one end on top of the other. This will allow us to balance and make use of our weight. This simulates exactly the same movement and tension. It's an incredible alternative for the.

Dollybells

The kettle-bell shoulders press is another important shoulder exercise. You can use either a dumbbell, or a kettlebell. The movement involves pushing the weight higher than your shoulder, keeping your abdomen tight, elbows slightly bent, and performing a slow, delicate motion. It is important to focus on the goal of hypertrophy when building shoulders. You don't want to push too much weight. Both men and woman look amazing with broad shoulders. Having the shoulder separated from the arm creates a visual of a V. This makes your waist look slimmer and your upper body stronger. A common mistake made by bodybuilders, especially young men is to only focus on the shoulder. The second major mistake is to not control your body fat. To achieve broad shoulders, one must have a low enough percentage of body fat to make the separation between the arms and the chest visible.

Otherwise, the incredible size and beauty this muscle has will remain invisible.

To ensure proportional development and growth of the triceps and triceps with high intensity pushups, the stress and tension they are subject to will be sufficient. To further disrupt the push day, pushing too many pushups will make the chest the most prominent muscle group. Esthetically, the triceps as well as the shoulders will experience growth, since your body needs to develop the muscles in a proportional way.

High triceps priority makes diamond pushups more effective at growing the arms' back. The shoulder muscles support the body while we pushups. The tension they produce will result in a growing of the shoulders. But, a great looking physique is not just about having proportionate shoulders. We want "beautiful" shoulders that are slightly larger then what our average anatomy would allow. To remedy this, we included shoulder exercises. We will use the same schedule as before. However, the two push day workouts will be different. The first will be focused on resistance while the other will concentrate on functionality. That means one day will have only 3 exercises to complete, while the other will have many more options and more complex execution. The workout program itself will be at the back of the book. It will include 3 workouts (for the resistance push day) and 3 for function day. You'll also find instructions on how you can combine them and increase difficulty.

Pull day

Pull day is your second training day. You will continue the same training method twice a week. Pull-ups are the most important exercises in this category. You may want to consider buying a pullup bar for your home. Most readers will struggle to perform more than one or two pullups.

To begin, you should do assisted pull-ups first. Then work your way upwards. This amazing exercise will make your back and biceps stronger.

These exercises include pull ups, assisted pullups and negative pulling ups. Yes, pull-ups only. This remarkable exercise stimulates back muscle growth and biceps development amazingly effectively. For extra tension, add an extra bicep exercise here and you have the perfect pull-up routine. Notice how these three exercises can be used to modify the pull-up. However, the difficulty of each variation is based on whether regular pull-ups will be too difficult at first. The assisted pull up will then be the preferred one. This routine can help increase strength. Additionally, the bicep also plays an important role in pulling off a pullup. You will notice growth in the arms soon. Calisthenics are the best method to build strength and muscles.

Assistive Pull-ups will need a band. These bands can be purchased in your nearest sports store. They are also quite affordable. These bands can be purchased in three different colors, depending on how strong they are. The red band is the best as it gives you the most leverage. As you train, wrap the band around one end of the bar. Insert your feet into the opposite end. Once the band is wrapped, have all your bodyweight fall on the band. Once the elastic is tensioned, you can hold your hands approximately 2 inches above the shoulders and then pull yourself upwards. This will engage the back and biceps. It is easy to do 8-12 repetitions with the assistance of the band.

If you're unable to pull-ups then the next exercise to work on your back is the negative pullups. It's an alternate that solves the problem of strength. The body will do all the work through resistance to gravity. This is called negative bodybuilding. You simply need to grab the bar and hold it while gravity pulls you downward. It's important to maintain your balance and resist gravity. The bar can be held by grabbing it and jumping on it. This will help keep your back muscles engaged and keeps you from bending over.

The ultimate goal of these exercises is to improve your strength in order to be able pull-ups more often. The classic pull up is the greatest back exercise. This activates the back, and biceps to increase growth. Due to its remarkable effectiveness, even professional bodybuilders use it on a frequent basis. A regular pull-up is the heart of any back workout.

If executed correctly, pull ups offer the best tension, flexion, and tension for the back and hips. Keep your shoulders as high at the bar as possible, and keep your hands under control. Do not do the pull-up abruptly. The effects of tension shrinking will cause the muscles to contract faster.

To complement the engagement and tension that have been exercised on the biiceps, the biceps curl can be used. A dumbbell of 5-12.5 kg. It is highly recommended that you use a dumbbell that weighs between 5 and 12,5 kg. A kettlebell, however, will be just as effective. You will need to start from a relaxed place, and then lift the dumbbells to the shoulders. This will help you flex your biceps, as well as engage the other muscles. You will see an increase in arm strength from the pull-ups. The bicep curl complements this. To simulate resistance with the resistance band, we will place one arm onto the band at a time and then use the other to generate resistance.

It is important to keep in mind that the term "big arms" does not refer only to the size of your biceps. In fact, big arms can also be attributed to the growth of your triceps. They account for approximately 1/3 of the arm's total size.

Leg Day

Leg day is one of the most important training days, even though it is not often appreciated. I include one leg day per semaine in my program and use only two exercises to strengthen the leg muscles. Simply stated, building leg muscles is essential for strength, calorie usage, and overall appearance. Some people are naturally gifted with strong calves and muscle legs. A person does not need huge quads to look balanced, but having some muscle adds a nice touch to everyone's appearance.

Begin with the squat. This classic exercise is used often by bodybuilders to activate the leg, and butt muscles. You will start by positioning your legs at shoulder width, with your toes in front. Slowly you will begin to lower, keeping your back straight. You must squat until the lines running from your knees to the ground and from the knee to your butt are 90 degrees. An arm extension can help with balance, especially in the beginning. You must also ensure that your heels are not lifted off the ground.

Squats can prove to be very efficient even with a trained individual. The high repetition rate can lead to soreness. As such, you should add weights.

Here is a demonstration of the squat, performed with both resistance bands and kettlebells.

Lunge is the next exercise to help develop the leg muscles. An online video with more details about the lunge's mechanics can be found. We are fairly confident that most people from high school know the Lunge. The lunge consists in taking one large step forward while keeping your back straight while your legs and legs stay tight.

Cardiovascular health and abs

Due to the popularity of 6 pack abs, more people will do more ab training in pursuit of that dream. Although visible abs may seem simple, it is actually much more difficult. The abdominal muscles must be trained to improve their size. However, if a person's body is very fat, the newly trained abs may not be visible. When trying to build a six-pack, the biggest mistake people make is to focus too much on training the muscles and not enough on nutrition and cardio. If you only want to have a small six pack, or if you already have low body fat, it may suffice to train the muscles, and not do any work to lower your body.

We decided to group cardio and abs under one heading as they go together. The goal is to get strong abs without having to do cardio and pay close attention to nutrition. But, once the muscles grow, you will have strong abs. The space between the abdominal squares will be filled with body fat which will make the real progress and effort much less apparent.

Start with the abs exercises. We only need to do two. To form the popular six-pack, the abdominal muscle we are after is the 6th square. So we have to train all 6 muscles. You will be doing this exercise twice, one for the upper and lower rows and one for the middle and lower. Begin with the sit-up and finish with the leg raise. They will both require repeated training. However, instead of overcomplicating training by doing many different exercises, and making it more difficult, we keep things simple and efficient. I have done ab training for years. I do 200 sit ups and 100 legs raises. They are enough to leave me feeling sore the next day. While you can train abs for up to 30 minutes per session it is not recommended. In 5-10 mins, you can do the same exercise twice without stopping. Sit-ups consist of lying down in a position with your knees bent. The upper body is on the back. The repetition is when your upper body is lifted approximately 45 degrees. This allows you to contract the abdominal muscle by putting your arms along-side or on the chest.

You do not have to go all up. But, you can get stronger abdominal muscles in the future. The second exercise will require you to lay on your back. To do this, raise your legs so that they are 90 degrees in front of your body. This will contract the abdominals by engaging the lower ab row.

I designed a cardio section that's both efficient, but didn't need to exhaust me or run a lot. I chose to apply the method I used to trim body fat over the past year. For 6 days I did cardio and ran the last day. These numbers will likely change for the first few days, with 2 days consisting of quick workouts lasting 10 minutes, and 1 day comprising a longer run.

You can choose to do knee taps, knee raises, or both for the first exercise.

Extremely easy, it involves placing your hands on the backside of your head or along side the torso and running in place with your knees raised. We'll discuss the details of how much and how often we do this in the next chapter when we talk to workout programs. It's enough to know that this is your best friend when it comes to fat-burning.

Finally, running is all that's needed.

Jump rope is an alternative to knee lifts. Jump rope is a fantastic way to increase endurance and burn fat. Boxers often train with it. If you're willing to learn the actual movement, which can be challenging for someone not familiar with jumping rope, I recommend switching the knee lifts to jump rope.

Chapter 9: The Science Of Weight Loss

It's strange to speak of "the science" of weight loss. Although it is scientific in nature, it also requires determination, perseverance, motivation, as well all other words that can be used to describe someone who wants to make positive changes in their lives. The good news is that I won't be using a lot scientific jargon to explain the intricacies of weight loss. (The use of words isn't important, but the understanding gained from the explanation is.

The truth is that all the cliche-ish advice you have heard about weight loss is true. "Eat less, exercise more," "Calories In, Calories Out," "Feel The Burn" and "Eat Clean." All these words matter. They are all true. They all work. Technically, you can eat junk food to lose weight if your calories are higher than your meals. Don't get too excited. You might look smaller, but your body would look exactly like the food that you ate. Food is what your body uses for energy. You'll end up feeling deprived and unable to eat healthy food.

The majority of this book will give you instructions on how to do different exercises, and even a schedule. This section is however going to show you everything you need in order to win the fights in the kitchen. Don't worry! You don't have to be a gourmet chef making complicated meals. It's up to your creativity and imagination to create complicated meals.

These are the most important points I want to emphasize about your diet. (Diet isn't a dirty word, though. It's simply used to delineate the food you eat every day. This word should not be feared.

Okay, we're off to the next:

Keep a daily journal. While it may seem time-consuming, it really can prove to be very beneficial. It will help you find your weak spots and strengths by keeping a log. Your food log will show you why you're not getting results you like or those you need. Although it's not necessary to follow the same routine indefinitely, it's a good idea to at least start. It wouldn't hurt to check in with your diet every now and again.

You should eat breakfast. It's not necessary to eat your breakfast immediately after you wake up. However, you don't want to wait too much. It is best to have breakfast within the first hour of awakening. Simple and quick meals are acceptable. Egg white eggs are quick and easy to make. You could also make oatmeal with berries. Or grab some fruit, nuts, and a protein smoothie. There are so many things you can do to make a healthy, nutritious breakfast. Even leftovers can be used for breakfast. Don't limit yourself. Look beyond the box.

Don't skip meals. If you want to lose weight or tone your body, skip meals. While it is an easy way for you to trim calories, you will end up paying big. Don't do it! If you are feeling hungry, eat! A meal doesn't need to be elaborate or contain only the finest foods. It's important to ensure the food has a high nutritional value.

Don't drink your calories. This is something that you have likely heard before. Water is essential to your body's proper functioning. You should drink the right amount. (Eight 8oz. This is a good place for a start. Additionally, water is a good way to make sure you don't consume unnecessary calories.

You can get around 120 calories from 6-8 oz. of your favorite orange juice. If you're like most people then you consume 2 to 3 glasses. Those calories add up quickly. You think you're drinking harmless juice, but it adds up quickly. You drink soda? It's exactly the same. Take into account the amount of sugar contained in each. Be aware of your choices. You should always choose plain water. If you like something a little more flavorful make sure to count the calories.

Make sure you eat enough protein. Protein is slow to digest, so you can keep your hunger at bay for longer. Your weight loss efforts are greatly improved if your metabolism is boosted. There are many ways to get enough healthy protein. There are many protein-rich foods, including beef, lambs, pork, turkeys, chicken and eggs. This list is not comprehensive, but it will give you an idea of what to eat. Protein shakes may be a good option for those who are in a hurry to meet their daily protein needs.

Carbs do not make the enemy. Contrary popular belief, carbohydrates don't make the devil's spawn. Overeating carbs can cause adverse reactions. Most people assume that "bad carbohydrates" are strictly prohibited. Carbohydrates can be good or evil, but that is not the truth. While some carbs might be more nutritious than others, they can all be good. Simple carbs primarily consist of sugars. They offer short bursts, but they can also make it difficult for people to lose weight. However, you don't need to have them. You will just need to watch your intake and pay attention to your body's reactions to them. It would be in your best interests to consume complex carbs, such foods made from whole grains, fruits, or vegetables.

These simple yet important guidelines will ensure you slim down. These are guidelines [not rules] and should not be followed exactly. However, it is important to keep to the basic suggestions within each of the guidelines. Take control of what you are eating and when. It doesn't have be a constant battle, but you should be conscious of your choices.

Chapter 10: The List Of Bodyweight Training Exercises

Please take some time to read through the instructions for each weight exercise. It will not only make a great use of your time, but also allow you to complete each exercise correctly. It's true: One good rep is better then five bad reps. Instead of doing MORE reps without good form, do less.

Consider making this your first ever casual workout. Take a look at the description and start doing 10 reps of each exercise. You will get about 240 total reps.

Push-ups

Place your hands flat on the ground, just below your shoulder joint. Now stretch out your body into a plank position, with your feet together. Core tightening is important. Now, bend your elbows to bring your chest down to the floor.

Reverse the direction. Now straighten your arms and push your body back into the original position. Keep your elbows as close together as possible to your body. If your elbows and shoulders feel sore from the early morning push-ups, then you can scale back to your knees and do the push ups from there. Don't be ashamed to increase your push-ups especially early in the day!

Shoulder Tap Push-ups

Keep going in the push-up position until the end. Then, you can balance by placing your bodyweight on the left arm. Next, raise your righthand off of the ground and touch your left side with your right. Perform a Push-up again and alternate sides.

Shoulder Rotation Pushups

Complete a Push-up in the top position. Then, support your left arm with your bodyweight and balance it on your right side. Now you can lift your right leg off the ground and reach towards the ceiling. You will be able to control your upper body and rotate your head to the right. Keep going at the top and continue to Push-up. You can also alternate the rotations on the opposite side.

Push-ups with Hand Release

Perform a normal Pushup. However, at the bottom, lower the weight of your whole body onto the floor. After that, lift your hands off to the surface for a second before moving back up to the starting place.

Front Planks - Elbows or hands

You can do the classic Push-up by placing your hands on ground below your shoulders. To finish, lower yourself to your elbows. You should not allow your back to arch towards the ground around your stomach and/or hips. This posture should last for 30 seconds. This is a similar, but slightly different position.

Side Planks; Left and Right; Elbows. Hands

Standing at the top of the Push up position, place your bodyweight upon your left arm. Next, use your balance to raise your righthand off the floor and place your right hand by your side. You should rotate your whole body so your right shoulder points towards the ceiling. Keep your legs straight and your right heel on the ground. Your core should be tightened as much as possible. Alternate the side. This position will last approximately 30 seconds. (Alternatively, you can lower yourself to your elbow for a slightly different effect.

Shoulder Touch Planks

Start in the Push-up pose with your hands below your shoulders. You can now shift your bodyweight and place your right elbow on your left shoulder. Next, bring your right leg up and tap your left shoulder. Continue on the opposite side. These should always be done slowly and with the proper tension. If you feel strong, push up between each pair of plank taps!

Shoulder Rotation Planks

In the Push-up position, get into the top position. Your bodyweight should be supported on your left arm. Now you need to balance and raise your right-hand off the floor. You will control your upper body's rotation to the right by bending your elbows. Keep going at the top of Push-ups and continue rotating the other side.

Sit ups

With your feet in front of you, place your feet on the earth. Then, place your back against the ground so your head touches the ground. Allow your hands to touch the floor with your fingertips. Let your arms swing towards your feet. Keep your head and body in line until your hands touch the ground. Continue doing this.

V-ups are also known as Jackknives

Lay flat on your back, with your knees bent and your heels in contact with the ground. Now stretch your hands so that your hands touch the ground behind you head. Then, swing your legs towards vertical and lift your upper body up so your hands touch the ground. To control the entire movement, make sure your legs are straight. Also, tension your core by keeping your spine tight. With your arms and legs extended, lower yourself back to the starting position.

Squats

Place your feet shoulder-width apart with your toes pointed slightly forward. Bend your knees and bring your upper body down towards your heels. Balance your balance with your arms by extending forward. Move down as low you are able to. Your butt should not touch your knees. You can push your upper back towards the beginning position by using your legs. You should keep your knees in front of you and not straight ahead. You are free to swing your arms if necessary to maintain a rhythm and balance.

Jumping Squats

Place your feet about shoulder-width apart with your toes slightly outwards. Bend your knees to bring your upper body down towards your heels. Then, use your arms and extend your arms outwards to balance. Move down as low and flexible as possible. Your butt should touch the floor slightly below your knees. Start by extending your legs and pushing your entire body off of the ground. After reaching the bottom, you will be able to raise your feet so that your feet are simultaneously up in the air. To maintain balance and rhythm, you can swing your arms to the side.

Standing Lunges

Standing straight up, keep your feet shoulder-width apart. Next, extend your left foot as far forward as you can. Keep your right hand in place by rolling your toes forward. To bring your right knee down to the ground, keep tension in you quads and use your arms to balance. Next, lift your body up using your left arm to return to the original position. Continue doing the same thing with the second leg.

Jumping Lunges

Continue to Lie on your left leg and lift your right leg off the ground. This is the point where you don't need to push yourself back (or walk forward as in Walking Lunges), but instead, you can JUMP to get into the right leg Lunge. Tension in your quads will help you control your descent into the last lunge position.

Jumping Jacks

Now stand upright with your feet together. Your hands should touch the outside of your thighs. You will now need to extend your feet so that your feet touch the ground. Once you're in this position, move your arms back into the starting position. This should all be done very quickly.

Jog at a Park

It says exactly what it means. Keep your legs straight and jog. While this is not the best way to replace a run, it makes a great filler for a home workout.

High Knees

Keep your feet approximately shoulder width apart. Now, raise your left leg so that your knees are parallel to the floor. Continue to alternate with your other leg. Repeat this several times, until you can run in place with your knees raised. Repeat this process with each leg.

Butt Kickers

Keep your feet approximately shoulder width apart. Your left foot should be lifted so that it touches your butt. Then repeat the process for the opposite leg. Do this in rapid succession. It should feel like running in a straight line and kicking your feet with your heels. Each leg should be counted as a rep.

Mountain Climbers

Start by putting your hands below your shoulders in the classic Pushup position. Your left foot should remain in this position. But, your right foot should be lifted so that your right knee touches the ground. Do the same with the other side. Alternate at very rapid speeds.

Burpees

Start by standing straight with your feet shoulder-width apart. Then, bend your knees so that your feet are about shoulder width apart. Now place your hands on to the floor in front. You will now be able to push your feet up behind you, and then lower your body so that it is just below the bottom of the Pushup position. Your chest should touch the floor. Then, move back up by pushing your upper-body off the floor using your arms. After reaching the top position in the Push-up, raise your back legs and reach the bottom position. Next, perform the famous burpee jump by jumping from the bottom position. Keep your feet on the ground at all times and keep your hands up high enough to reach your head. Burpees is a fantastic and terrible sport!

Tuck jumps

Place your feet shoulder-width apart on a straight, upright position. Move your hips and knees forward to "load" the spring. Then, jump as high you can. Keep your hips and knees bent as you jump so your legs are as close as possible to your chest.

Glute Bridges

Lay flat on your stomach on the ground with your arms in front of you and your palms facing the floor. Bend your knees to lift your feet off the ground. This is your starting point. Push your butt towards the floor, so that your knees meet your hips. Try to push your hips as high and straight as you can. For stability, you should keep your arms, hands and soles of your shoes on the flooring. To return to your starting position, lower the butt as soon as you reach this height.

Inch Worm (also know as Walk Out)

Place your feet about shoulder width apart on a flat surface. Your hands should be pointing down towards the ground, as if your hamstrings were being stretched. Place your hands palms down on the floor in front of you feet. Then, gradually shift your weight away from your legs to your arms. Keep moving forward slowly with your hands until your hands reach the classic push-up position. You will then be able to reverse the direction of your "walking" hands so that you are back at the starting point.

Chair Dips

Place the chair against a wall. Position the back of the chair towards the wall. As you turn your back towards the chair, place both your hands on its edge. Then, stretch your legs straight in front and away from the chair. As you get out of this position, lower your body as low as possible by bending your arms. You should try to drop as low as possible. Now, get back to your starting position.

Chapter 11: Workout

1 Minute Jumproe

1 Minute Push Ups

1 Minute Mountain Climbers.

1 Minute Burpees

Important

Take no breaks between each exercise.

Recover for two minutes after completing the cycle.

Repeat the whole cycle 2 more times.

The entire workout lasts for 10 minutes.

1m+1m+1m+1m =4 min

2m = 2 minutes

1m+1m+1m+1m =4 min

Total = 10 Minutes

Jumprope, One-Minute

If you're looking to lose weight quickly (around 200 calories in just a few minutes), then this supplement is for you.

This is what you get when rope hopping works:

*Your muscles, including the quadriceps (gastrocnemius), quadriceps (hamstrings), glutes/gastrointestinal, stomach, lower arm, and deltoids-get some exercise.

*You will feel more confident and ready to work with others.

*Rope-bouncing is an excellent way to build solid bones.

Be careful if your knees feel weak or awkward. Bouncing rope is easy to master and can really help your joints.

Getting started.

The most important piece is a good jump rope. A plastic beaded, or divided rope is better for performance and durability. This rope weighs in at about half-pound. The rope swings easily and is powerful enough to provide force.

Tips and techniques

Rope hopping has a unique advantage: you don't need to know a lot about rigging or follow a specific route. With a fast exercise, great structure, some thought, and a few tips to keep it simple, you can easily lose weight and tone your body. These tips will get your started.

Good form is key. Jumping is easier and fun when you are in good form.

The components of the leap look like this.

The twirl.

Keep your elbows in line with your body. Your shoulders should be down and your chest area steady. Turn the rope by bringing your hands to your hips.

The jump.

Rope-hopping is not an exaggerated effect movement. The rope should be bounced as high and as far as you feel comfortable.

During the whole activity, keep your knees slightly bent.

Do a "ropeless" warmup.

Warm up with a few minutes walking, strolling, and exercises before you start skipping. Your muscles will become more sensitive to bouncing and you will have sharper reflexes.

Cushion your landing.

If you were a child, it was perfectly safe. Your adult hips, knees, and hips tilt toward a more cushioned landing place. A low covering, hardwood floors, or blacktop make for more secure surfaces.

Keep the beat.

Jumping rope with upbeat music encourages creativity and makes it more like playing. Turn up your favorite tune and jump to it. Rope hopping is a freestyle movement that can be achieved with great music.

Run, skip, jump.

The greatest hop rope move is a simple two-footed bounce each whirl. It is whirl., bounce., spin., jump. You're not secured in the two-advancebout. These moves mix it up but also make it easier for your body to move longer without taking a rest.

Single-foot jumps

You can substitute jumping with one foot. To do checks of one- to three jumps each side, bounce both feet.

Heel kicks

You should fix one leg with each bounce and then contact the heel. Substitute the other leg.

One-Minute Pushups

Push-ups, when we think about bodyweight, are one of the most effective exercises to strike a chord.

It doesn't get any simpler than pressing your body up and putting your fingers on the ground.

If you begin the development, you will be able to tell if the quality of your chest is satisfactory. There are many benefits to properly performing the push-up regardless of how simple the idea may seem.

Proper positioning.

Correctly performing push-ups will ensure that your muscles work! Push-ups will work your chest, shoulders, arms and chest. You will also be using your abdominals and back muscles when doing push-ups.

Push-Up hand position

You can strengthen your wrists and stretch them before developing wrist problems.

Keep your hands close to your shoulders. Spread your thumbs so that your thumbs touch your shoulders. Although this may require some adjustments for comfort, the spacing isn't too tight or too wide.

Push-up Elbow Position

Place your elbow parallel to your middle finger. You should draw a straight line from your elbow to your middle finger.

As you align your elbows, bring your elbows to your sides.

The best way to strengthen your shoulder and increase your health is to align your joints correctly.

The Push-Up.

Keep your body rigid and tight to perform a push-up.

When you keep your posture straight, the push-up will go smoothly if you are able to lower your body.

Push straight up and downward while holding your lower body tightly so your whole body moves in one direction. Your shoulders, back, hips and hips should all move together.

One-minute Mountain Climbers.

Mountain climbers are an excellent way to increase your cardiovascular fitness and muscle strength. Mountain climbers perform in plank posture. This means that you slowly raise one knee under your body. This is similar to running, but you are also holding your whole body in the air, which makes it more difficult and engages more muscles.

Mountain climbers are good for your cardio and strength. Your arms are involved as you need to balance your body and keep your knees in place while you swing your knees.

Proper form.

Begin in a push up position. With your arms about shoulder-width and your body and legs straight, you will be in a push up position. Quickly bring one leg under your body and do a jump motion. As fast as you can, switch your legs. Keep one leg straight, the other bent under your body. Your legs should feel like you are lifting them off the ground. Start slow if this is your first time doing it. Gradually increase your speed (just like running), and your knees will travel more distance.

Common Mistakes

Your hips should be elevated when you bring your knee into the ground.

Your arms should not be too far out or in front.

Muscles Worked.

You will strengthen your core muscles (abs, buttocks, quadriceps & hamstrings) during exercise.

One-Minute Burpees

Burpees will make you feel completely exhausted after just a few burpees.

Instructions

Begin in an squat position. Keep your hands on the floors.

Place your feet in a push-up position.

Now return your feet directly to the squat.

As high as possible, extend your arms from the squat.

Burpees should be performed one after the next to enjoy the many benefits that this activity has to offer.

Do More.

You can also make the burpees a bit more difficult by using some basic variations. To make your burpees faster or more difficult, you can include an applaud pull-up.

American Fitness Magazine recommends a harder variation. At the end, you should bounce up to grab a draw down bar. After performing a pushup, lower down and perform another burpee.

Chapter 12: How to Ensure Your Safety and Get Fast Results

Are you looking to find additional tips that will increase safety, avoid injury, and provide quick results when you exercise? This chapter will help you. These guidelines provide additional guidance to help ensure your safety while you are working out and that you achieve the desired results as quickly as possible.

For 5-10 min, warm up prior to your workout and cool down.

Start slow and slowly increase your activity.

If you're unable or unwilling to train, it is best not to do so. Overuse of certain sports such as tennis (elbows), walking (feet, knees, ankles), and swimming can lead to damage to specific body parts. Avoid injuries by mixing different activities and getting enough sleep.

Be attentive to your body. Watch out for signs and cues. You should not exercise if your body is feeling very tired or sick. If you feel like you're going to faint or feel that you have constant pains and aches, reduce the time. Your body needs to be observed so that you know when it's time for rest.

When you're doing strength training, don't lose your good form. Do not compromise your form to get sets or reps done quickly, or to struggle to lift heavy loads.

Avoid intense workouts in hot and humid environments. If the temperature exceeds 70 degrees F, you should slow down.

Do not stick with the exact same routine - As a beginner, you may make the common mistake of repeating the same exercise routine every day. Your muscles should not become accustomed. Mix it up with your workouts. Vary your intensity and time. You can train on the elliptical bike or on a bicycle one day, and then on a treadmill on the next. Then, you can go for a walk outside the next morning.

Be sure to set goals once in a while. This is why you should set new goals occasionally. This will motivate you to work out every day.

You can try new things and do different routines. Something new is needed to challenge your workout habits. Seek out activities that require movement. Engaging in something new can help you avoid getting bored, losing focus, and losing motivation.

Be aware that numbers are not everything. You can gain invaluable feedback by keeping track of your running speed or heart rate. But if you are obsessive about using these trackers, you can reduce the excitement and enjoyment that you get from your chosen physical activity. You might even feel more confident if you don't feel 100% well on a given day.

The trackers are great, but it is important to remember to unplug them when you get bored. You can then focus on what your body says. It is better to exercise at a pace that makes your body feel good than it is stressing you out. Listen to your body to ensure that you have a great workout.

Chapter 13: Other Tips for a Full Blast Home Workout

Amp your endurance

Work from home doesn't mean you aren't serious about your fitness routine as a gym member. Increase your aerobic endurance with intervals. This can be accomplished by following this strategy: high intensity exercise followed with low intensity recovery. You'll be able to burn more calories as well as train your body harder.

Example:

Week 1 – Strength exercises for 20 seconds and rest for 40 seconds

Week 2 - 30 second work, 30 second rest

Week 3 – 40 Seconds of Work, 20 Seconds Rest Interval

Power skips

The power skips can be used to enhance agility. This can be done 3 times per week. Just make sure you are moving as high as possible. While raising your right knee to about hip height, keep your left foot straight. Repeat the process with each leg.

Balance improvement

This is known by the modified-tree pose. Start by standing and then place your left heel on your right inner knee. Your arms should be extended overhead. Close your eyes. You want to keep your form as clean and simple as possible.

The Plank

If ab crunches feel too hard, you might try the planking pose. Tend to this position for at most 30 seconds. Your body should remain in one straight line from shoulders down to feet. This position is for enhancing your mid-section. Because your body would need to be steady, you should engage your glutes.

Flexibility is key

Weak glutes? It's easy to get stronger glutes! These exercises can be done at-home three times per week to increase your strength. Start by lying down on your stomach with your feet flattening on the ground. Your right knee should be pulled towards your chest by pulling your right hand toward your chest. By pushing your left foot into your left shoe, lift your hips. Continue to hold the position for 5 second and then turn your back.

Alternate your daily exercise routine

Every other day, move your entire body. It is important to have a designated day to work on upper body and the next day for lower-body exercises.

Remember:

The following tips are important when weight training

Start with a lighter body weight. Do not rush to lift heavier plates. You'll only cause injury to yourself.

Take a deep breath as you lift the weights. Then exhale as your return to the starting point in a controlled, slow way.

Even if the machine is brand new, it is important to carefully read any warning signs or stickers before operating it.

Do not lift weights without securing the collars on the plates.

To reduce muscle soreness, perform each exercise with more reps but at lighter weight. You must also stretch your muscles at the end of each exercise.

Children should not have access to dumbbells and any other exercise equipment. Remember that you are exercising at home. You should always be cautious to avoid unpleasant situations.

Chapter 14: Rowers

A rower (or a machine that can row) is used to increase stamina. It also helps with upper body strength and endurance. A handle is typically attached to a flywheel and has a cable. It works by pulling the handle toward your chest while your legs are straightened. The seat then glides backward, mimicking the act of rowing.

A rowing system usually has a foot stretcher along with a rail to allow for the seat to glide. There is also a handle attached that controls the flywheel. A rowing machine may be an alternative for running or walking. It can be a great way to reach your fitness goals, because it builds, tone and strengthens your muscles and helps you burn calories.

Benefits

This improves the heart, lung function and circulation.

Low-impact workout that targets legs, hips, buttocks, and back with each step.

These exercises are effective for toning the muscles and burning calories.

Rowing is often regarded as one of most beneficial forms of exercise.

Average Calories Burned

Harvard Health Publications estimates that a one-hour intense workout by a 185-pound individual on the rowing machines can burn 377 calories. According to an American College of Sports Medicine publication, a 155-pound person exercising at moderate intensity can burn 493 calories each hour.

Price Range

The most expensive rowing machines are priced between $900-$1,250. But there are models that start at $180-$400. It is important to compare all options.

Different Types Of Rowers

Air Resistance Rowing Machines

The air resistance rowing machine has a large flywheel that houses a fan blade. The fan turns when the handle is pulled, which generates wind resistance. The speed and force with which you pull on the handlebar will increase resistance.

Piston Resistance Rowing Machines

The piston resistance device has two hydraulic pistons which attach to the handle bars. The pistons allow for manual adjustment of the resistance. This type is typically less expensive than others.

Machines for water resistance rowing

This rower uses an anti-slip water tank. The water used to resist makes it the most realistic type of rower.

Magnetic Resistance Rowing machines

Electromagnets can generate resistance. It becomes difficult to find momentum because the flywheel is slowed by the magnets.

Things to Consider before Buying a Rower

Goals and intensity

Take into account your goals when choosing the right type and model of rowing machines for you. A low-cost, lightweight rowing machine with moderate resistance is ideal if your goal is to lose weight. To increase your intensity and build strength, you might want to look at rowing machines that have higher tension levels.

Screen

The LCD screen should display useful information such as distance and speed. These numbers are very important to people, and can be used to monitor their heart rate.

Space

Also, think about the space in your home. The magnetic or water resistance rowing equipment is not foldable, so they are less portable than the others. You will find lighter and compact rowers. You will need enough space to do the rower motions.

Position adjustable

To avoid injury, the user must always be in the right position for rowing. You should adjust the distance between seat and handle bars.

Rowing machines, although often overlooked, are my favorite form of exercise. They can work a lot on your body, tone muscles better than any other type of equipment, and they burn a lot calories.

Chapter 15: Sitting & Standing Band Exercises

Like every other chapter, we will be discussing exercises for bands that involve sitting or standing.

* Resistance Band Therapy For Ankle Flexion Exercise

To start, wrap a loop of resistance around an anchored platform. (Tie one end of loop to the anchor).

You can take a seat in a chair, and then sit straight up on it.

Place one end of the band on the ankle of your leg, while straightening the other.

Place your head in a relaxed position on the chair rest. Swing your leg in a forward or backward direction for a few seconds.

Gently return your toes and swing them gently around your knee.

For as long and as you feel comfortable, continue the exercise.

The Lateral Band walks with The Resistance Band.

Make sure you tie a loop resistant band around your waistline.

So that your feet are at an appropriate distance, you can create tension around the resistance band.

Place your left leg in a semi-squat position.

Start by moving your right foot in a sideways direction. Then, move your left leg in the opposite direction. Finally, move your right foot inside the other.

Continue to do these exercises as often as possible until you are comfortable.

* The Standing Abduction Exercise.

Attach any therapy bracelet that is loop enabled to your leg and anchor it.

Your left side should be facing the anchor platform.

Fix the right ankle to your resistance band.

Move your right leg up a bit above the ground in an effort to produce tension.

You can raise your left leg by taking a slow, steady note and contracting your muscle hips. When you're doing this, ensure that you have a good support platform nearby.

You may return to your initial position. Perhaps in seconds, or even minutes.

* Sit-Abduction Resistance Band Exercise

Grab a chair, and then sit down.

You can place a loop resistance therapy bracelet around your left or right legs just above your knees.

Gently spread your feet and slowly move your knees inwards.

Make sure to rotate your legs before you separate them.

Keep your legs straight for a time, preferably for several seconds. After that, you can move in a stilled position and then put your knees back together.

You might want to try these again.

* Concentration Curl Resistance Band Therapy Exercise For Arms

Standing straight up, bring your right side to the front. Then, place the middle portion of the resistance underneath your right foot (foot).

Keep one end of therapy band in your other hand, and then relax your arm elbow to the inside portion of your knee.

You can place your palms slightly away from your knees. Next, fold your resistance bands up and snuggle your biceps in your hands.

Gently relax your spine and return to your old position.

Keep repeating these steps until you reach the desired time.

* The Standing Biceps Curling - Resistance Band Therapy

Keep your legs straight and place your feet on top of the resistance band.

You should hold both handles with both hands. Your hands should be in a relaxed position.

You can hold your band by holding your hand and placing it in your palm so that your palm fingers face you.

Pull your arm up, and it will pull up the resistance band.

Pull in until your pull is close to your shoulders.

This will either create or cause a tightening effect on the biceps.

Move your head a little to the side, just below your shoulder level to experience the benefits of the exercise on your biceps.

Keep going until you feel comfortable.

* Triceps Kickback Resistance Band Exercise.

Keep your head straight.

Keep your right leg straight in front.

Place your resistance band beneath your feet. Now, hold your hands in your hands and keep your palms towards you.

Your elbows bend along with you as you raise resistance band handles.

While holding onto the resistance band handles with your hands, extend your arms outwards and keep your hands in place.

To release tension from the band, relax your arms.

* Resistance Band Overhead Triceps Training.

Get a tube resist band for sitting or standing upright.

Place the band in the middle under your hip and place the chair on top.

As you grasp the band handles on your both hands, raise your hands.

Place your elbows on your back so that your hands are bent at the elbows. Tension the band all the while.

Keep your arms straight and extend your arms out straight to make a parallel line to the ground. This position should be held for at least a few minutes or longer (or as long and hard as possible).

You can continue the exercise by repeating what was just said.

* The Kneeling Crunch Exercise

Attach a resistance strap to the top end of an anchor plate that is high.

134

Now, get down to kneeling.

While you are kneeling, wrap the resistance band around your shoulders. Now stretch your arms out.

When performing this exercise, you should be able to use your hips as well as your muscular abs.

Some people will bend over the resistance band to do this, while others may even bend along with it.

Continue the same procedure as before if you are comfortable doing more rounds.

* Wood-Chopper Resistance Band Therapy Exercise

A tubed resistance band should be purchased.

Anchor your resistance bands to a support structure that is high enough for the band anchor.

Now, move your hands over the support. Take the other end that isn't anchored with both of your arms. Do a good stretch up to your head.

Drag down the resistance band from your chest to your knees in a horizontal motion. This will allow you to rotate your hips backwards and keep your feet spinning.

Gently return to the original position after you've completed the exercise.

* Anti-Rotation Walkout Resistance Band Therapy.

Take a tubed resistance piece and anchor it just below the support.

Grab your free end of resistance band.

Get into a squatting position and show some tautness towards the band.

Keep your arms straight and hold on to your resistance. Your hips should be firmly clenched.

To stretch the band, move sideways from the anchor.

You can keep repeating the above steps for as many as you wish.

* Reversed Crunch Resistance Band Therapy Exercise

You should anchor your resistance band onto a support system, but you support platform should be at low ebb.

You will need to lie on your stomach with your face towards ceiling.

As you sit on the ground, elevate your knees until you are able to squat.

Put your resistance band around your toes.

You can also pull the band together with your feet for some band tautness.

You can continue pulling the band by keeping your abdominal muscles tight.

Keep going until you feel satisfied.

* The Bent Over Row Resistance Band Therapy Exercise.

As if you were going to squat, place your feet in front.

Don't resist and let your band slip under your feet.

Place your resistance bands handles on your arms straightening towards your hips.

Pull until your elbows form a right angle (90 degrees). The areas that feel the greatest impact from this exercise are your hip bones, back bones, and shoulder bones.

For multiple times, you can repeat the steps/procedures outlined above.

Conclusion

I hope you found Weight Training For Weight Loss beneficial and were able discover some very effective methods to lose weight.

The next step is to put what you have learned into practice and perform these exercises. However, I caution you to be patient. You can always go up later. You'll see your fat deposits disappear quickly if you add some aerobics to your weight training.

I appreciate your kind words and wish you the very best of luck.

www.ingramcontent.com/pod-product-compliance
Lightning Source LLC
Chambersburg PA
CBHW050731030426
42336CB00012B/1515